GALLBLADDER CANCER COOKBOOK

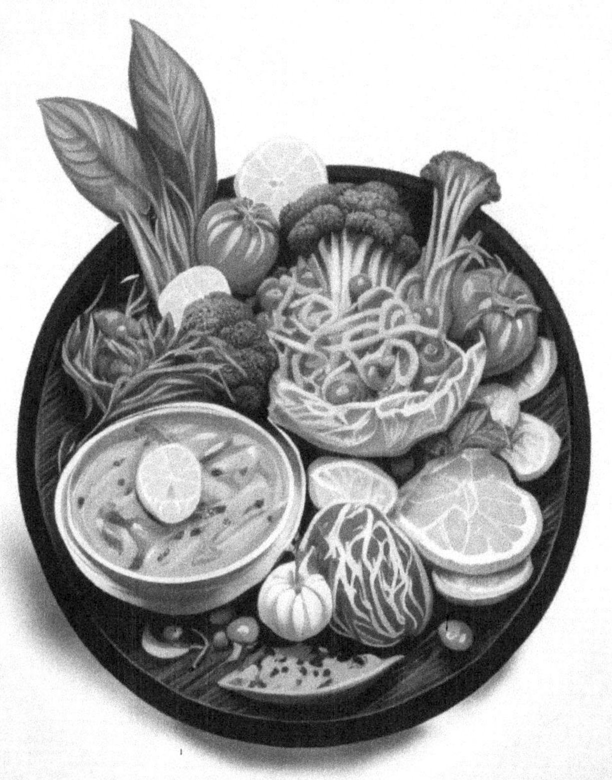

GET READY, LET'S FIGHT!

THIS BOOK BELONGS TO

Gallbladder Cancer Cookbook

==============================

Feeding Hope, Nurturing Health

Jetta Harlow Olson

Attribution: The resources utilized to design this cover were obtained from pexels.com.

ISBN: 9798868302909

Imprint: Independently Published

Disclaimer

This book's instructions, recommendations, or methods are not intended to replace professional medical guidance, diagnosis, or care. The information in this book is only meant to be used for educational purposes; it should not be used as a replacement for professional medical advice from a healthcare provider.

The authors and publisher of this book disclaim any responsibility for any negative effects or outcomes attributable to the use of the knowledge, suggestions, or methods offered in this book. Readers should speak with their doctor before beginning any new health or wellness program.

Despite the fact that the knowledge and research upon which the information in this book is based is up-to-date, medical procedures and recommendations may alter over time.

It is advised that readers seek out additional information and keep current with healthcare trends.

The authors' views are the only ones that are expressed in this book; they do not necessarily represent the publisher's views. The authors and publisher do not endorse or recommend any companies, items, or services that are mentioned in this book.

Despite making every effort to ensure the accuracy and comprehensiveness of the information in this book, the authors and publisher make no promises or representations of any kind, either explicitly or implicitly, regarding the information's suitability, reliability, or availability.

Any risks associated with relying on the information in this book are assumed by the reader.

Contents

Personal Motivation for the Cookbook 10
1.   GRILLED SALMON WITH LEMON AND HERBS 12
2.   QUINOA AND VEGETABLE STIR-FRY 13
3.   CHICKEN AND VEGETABLE SOUP 14
4.   BAKED SWEET POTATOES WITH GREEK YOGURT 15
5.   VEGETABLE AND LENTIL STEW 16
6.   SPINACH AND BERRY SALAD WITH GRILLED CHICKEN 17
7.   MASHED CAULIFLOWER WITH GARLIC AND HERBS 18
8.   TURKEY AND VEGETABLE SKEWERS 19
9.   AVOCADO AND BLACK BEAN SALAD 20
10.   OVEN-BAKED COD WITH LEMON AND HERBS 21
11.   LENTIL AND VEGETABLE CURRY 22
12.   EGG AND VEGETABLE WRAP 23
13.   CUCUMBER AND CHICKPEA SALAD 24
14.   TURKEY AND VEGETABLE QUINOA BOWL 25
15.   BAKED APPLES WITH CINNAMON AND WALNUTS 26
16.   SALMON AND ASPARAGUS FOIL PACKETS 27
17.   CAULIFLOWER RICE STIR-FRY WITH SHRIMP 28
18.   GREEK YOGURT PARFAIT WITH BERRIES AND ALMONDS 29
19.   CHICKPEA AND VEGETABLE STIR-FRY 30
20.   MANGO AND AVOCADO SALSA WITH GRILLED CHICKEN 31
21.   BAKED CHICKEN AND VEGETABLE CASSEROLE 32
22.   CAPRESE SALAD WITH BALSAMIC GLAZE 33
23.   PUMPKIN AND LENTIL SOUP 34
24.   SAUTÉED SPINACH WITH GARLIC AND PINE NUTS 35
25.   SWEET POTATO AND BLACK BEAN HASH 36
26.   TURKEY AND QUINOA STUFFED BELL PEPPERS 37
27.   MUSHROOM AND SPINACH FRITTATA 38
28.   ROASTED BRUSSELS SPROUTS WITH CRANBERRIES AND PECANS
      39
29.   TUNA AND WHITE BEAN SALAD 40
30.   CINNAMON-BAKED APPLES WITH GREEK YOGURT 41
31.   LEMON GARLIC SHRIMP WITH ZUCCHINI NOODLES 42
32.   QUINOA AND BLACK BEAN STUFFED PEPPERS 43
33.   TURMERIC AND GINGER CARROT SOUP 44
34.   BALSAMIC GLAZED CHICKEN WITH ROASTED VEGETABLES 45
35.   MANGO COCONUT CHIA PUDDING 46

36. BROCCOLI AND QUINOA CASSEROLE 47
37. ZESTY LEMON BASIL CHICKEN...48
38. SPAGHETTI SQUASH WITH TOMATO AND BASIL SAUCE 49
39. STUFFED PORTOBELLO MUSHROOMS 50
40. CHILLED BERRY SOUP 51
41. BAKED COD WITH MEDITERRANEAN SALSA...........................52
42. CAULIFLOWER AND BROCCOLI GRATIN...................................53
43. LEMON GARLIC ROASTED CHICKEN THIGHS..........................54
44. QUINOA SALAD WITH ROASTED VEGETABLES 55
45. MINTY WATERMELON SALAD 56
46. SESAME GINGER TOFU STIR-FRY...57
47. MANGO AND AVOCADO QUINOA SALAD 58
48. HONEY MUSTARD GLAZED SALMON 60
49. CABBAGE AND APPLE SLAW..61
50. DARK CHOCOLATE AND BERRY PARFAIT.................................62
51. LEMON HERB QUINOA WITH ROASTED VEGETABLES.................63
52. CILANTRO LIME CHICKEN SKEWERS 64
53. ROASTED GARLIC MASHED CAULIFLOWER 65
54. BLACK BEAN AND CORN SALSA...66
55. PEACH AND BERRY SMOOTHIE BOWL 67
56. SALMON AND ASPARAGUS FOIL PACKETS..............................68
57. QUINOA AND BLACK BEAN STUFFED SWEET POTATOES 69
58. GREEK CHICKEN SALAD WRAPS 70
59. CUCUMBER AVOCADO GAZPACHO 71
60. ALMOND BUTTER AND BANANA OVERNIGHT OATS 72
61. TURKEY AND VEGETABLE STIR-FRY 73
62. CAPRESE SALAD WITH GRILLED CHICKEN..............................74
63. MISO-GLAZED EGGPLANT WITH QUINOA 75
64. PESTO ZOODLES WITH CHERRY TOMATOES.............................76
65. BERRY AND SPINACH SMOOTHIE..77
66. LENTIL AND VEGETABLE CURRY...78
67. CAULIFLOWER AND CHICKPEA TACOS....................................80
68. MUSHROOM AND SPINACH QUICHE......................................81
69. SWEET POTATO AND BLACK BEAN BUDDHA BOWL....................82
70. COCONUT CHIA SEED PUDDING WITH MANGO.........................84
71. SPINACH AND FETA STUFFED CHICKEN BREAST.......................85
72. ROASTED VEGETABLE AND QUINOA STUFFED BELL PEPPERS 86
73. LEMON GARLIC SHRIMP WITH BROCCOLI.................................87
74. AVOCADO AND CHICKPEA SALAD 88
75. BANANA AND ALMOND BUTTER SMOOTHIE 90

76. MEDITERRANEAN QUINOA SALAD....................................91
77. TERIYAKI TOFU STIR-FRY 92
78. CABBAGE AND APPLE QUINOA SALAD........................93
79. LEMON HERB BAKED SALMON 95
80. GREEN SMOOTHIE BOWL..96

Personal Motivation for the Cookbook

As the creator of this cookbook, my personal motivation stems from a deep understanding of the challenges faced by individuals with Gallbladder Cancer. Witnessing the impact of this diagnosis on individuals and their loved ones inspired the creation of a resource that extends beyond the kitchen.

Cooking, at its core, is an expression of love and care. When faced with health challenges, it becomes a powerful tool for nourishment, healing, and a source of comfort. Through "Gallbladder Cancer Cookbook," my aim is to provide not just recipes, but a companion on your path—a guide filled with flavors that bring joy, and ingredients that support your well-being.

1. **Nutrient-Packed Healing:** Every recipe in this cookbook is carefully curated to include ingredients that are not only delicious but also chosen for their healing properties. From antioxidant-rich fruits to anti-inflammatory herbs, each bite is designed to contribute to your well-being.

2. **Simple and Accessible:** I understand the importance of simplicity, especially during challenging times. The recipes are crafted to be easy to prepare, with readily available ingredients, ensuring that cooking remains an enjoyable and manageable part of your routine.

3. **Dietary Tailoring:** Recognizing the unique dietary needs that come with Gallbladder Cancer, the

recipes provide options for customization. Whether you're managing specific dietary restrictions or seeking variety, these recipes are adaptable to your individual needs.

4. **Emotional Support:** Beyond the kitchen, "Gallbladder Cancer Cookbook" offers words of encouragement, tips for self-care, and stories of strength. It's a reminder that you're not alone on this journey, and every step you take toward nourishing your body is a victory.

In creating this cookbook, my hope is that it serves as a source of inspiration, comfort, and empowerment. May these recipes bring joy to your table, strength to your body, and warmth to your spirit. Remember, each meal is a celebration of life, a gesture of self-love, and a testament to the incredible strength within you.

Important Note: These recipes offer a variety of nutrient-rich ingredients and cater to different dietary preferences. Remember to tailor the portion sizes and ingredients to suit individual needs and dietary restrictions. Always consult with a healthcare professional before making significant changes to a patient's diet, especially for individuals undergoing Gallbladder Cancer treatment.

1. Grilled Salmon with Lemon and Herbs

Ingredients:

- 4 salmon fillets
- 2 tablespoons olive oil
- 1 lemon (juiced)
- 2 tablespoons fresh herbs (such as dill, parsley, or chives)
- Salt and pepper to taste

Instructions:

1. Preheat the grill.
2. In a small bowl, mix olive oil, lemon juice, and chopped herbs.
3. Brush the salmon fillets with the mixture and sprinkle with salt and pepper.
4. Grill the salmon for about 4-5 minutes on each side or until cooked through.

2. Quinoa and Vegetable Stir-Fry

Ingredients:

- 1 cup quinoa

- 2 cups mixed vegetables (broccoli, bell peppers, carrots)

- 2 tablespoons low-sodium soy sauce

- 1 tablespoon sesame oil

- 1 teaspoon grated ginger

- 2 cloves garlic (minced)

Instructions:

1. Cook quinoa according to package instructions.

2. In a large pan, stir-fry the mixed vegetables in sesame oil until slightly tender.

3. Add ginger and garlic, continue to stir-fry for 1-2 minutes.

4. Mix in cooked quinoa and soy sauce, stir until well combined.

3. Chicken and Vegetable Soup

Ingredients:

- 1 lb boneless, skinless chicken breast
- 8 cups low-sodium chicken broth
- 2 carrots, sliced
- 2 celery stalks, chopped
- 1 cup green beans, chopped
- 1 cup brown rice or rice noodles
- Fresh herbs (parsley or dill)
- Salt and pepper to taste

Instructions:

1. In a large pot, bring chicken broth to a simmer.
2. Add chicken breast and cook until done.
3. Remove chicken, shred it, and return it to the pot.
4. Add carrots, celery, green beans, and rice/noodles. Simmer until vegetables are tender.
5. Season with salt and pepper, sprinkle fresh herbs before serving.

4. Baked Sweet Potatoes with Greek Yogurt

Ingredients:

- 4 medium-sized sweet potatoes
- 1 cup Greek yogurt
- 1 tablespoon honey
- Cinnamon for sprinkling

Instructions:

1. Preheat the oven to 400°F (200°C).
2. Wash and prick sweet potatoes with a fork. Bake for about 45-60 minutes or until tender.
3. In a bowl, mix Greek yogurt and honey.
4. Once sweet potatoes are done, split them open, fluff the insides with a fork, and top with the Greek yogurt mixture.
5. Sprinkle with cinnamon before serving.

5. Vegetable and Lentil Stew

Ingredients:

- 1 cup dry lentils (rinsed)

- 4 cups vegetable broth

- 1 onion, chopped

- 2 carrots, diced

- 2 celery stalks, chopped

- 1 can diced tomatoes

- 2 cloves garlic, minced

- 1 teaspoon cumin

- 1 teaspoon turmeric

- Salt and pepper to taste

Instructions:

1. In a large pot, combine lentils, vegetable broth, onion, carrots, celery, tomatoes, garlic, cumin, turmeric, salt, and pepper.

2. Bring to a boil, then reduce heat and simmer for 25-30 minutes or until lentils are tender.

6. Spinach and Berry Salad with Grilled Chicken

Ingredients:

- 2 boneless, skinless chicken breasts

- 6 cups fresh spinach leaves

- 1 cup mixed berries (strawberries, blueberries, raspberries)

- 1/4 cup feta cheese, crumbled

- 1/4 cup balsamic vinaigrette dressing

Instructions:

1. Grill chicken breasts until fully cooked.

2. In a large bowl, toss fresh spinach, mixed berries, and crumbled feta.

3. Slice grilled chicken and place on top of the salad.

4. Drizzle with balsamic vinaigrette dressing before serving.

7. Mashed Cauliflower with Garlic and Herbs

Ingredients:

- 1 head cauliflower, chopped into florets

- 2 cloves garlic, minced

- 2 tablespoons olive oil

- 1/4 cup fresh herbs (parsley, chives)

- Salt and pepper to taste

Instructions:

1. Steam or boil cauliflower until tender.

2. In a blender or food processor, combine cauliflower, minced garlic, olive oil, and herbs.

3. Blend until smooth, season with salt and pepper.

8. Turkey and Vegetable Skewers

Ingredients:

- 1 lb lean ground turkey
- 1 zucchini, sliced
- 1 bell pepper, cut into chunks
- 1 red onion, quartered
- 2 tablespoons olive oil
- 1 teaspoon Italian seasoning
- Salt and pepper to taste

Instructions:

1. Preheat the grill or oven.
2. In a bowl, mix ground turkey with Italian seasoning, salt, and pepper. Shape into small meatballs.
3. Thread turkey meatballs onto skewers alternating with zucchini, bell pepper, and red onion.
4. Brush skewers with olive oil and grill or bake until turkey is cooked through.

9. Avocado and Black Bean Salad

Ingredients:

- 2 avocados, diced

- 1 can black beans, drained and rinsed

- 1 cup corn kernels (fresh or frozen)

- 1 red onion, finely chopped

- 1/4 cup cilantro, chopped

- Juice of 2 limes

- Salt and pepper to taste

Instructions:

1. In a large bowl, combine diced avocados, black beans, corn, red onion, and cilantro.

2. Squeeze lime juice over the salad and toss gently.

3. Season with salt and pepper before serving.

10.Oven-Baked Cod with Lemon and Herbs

Ingredients:

- 4 cod fillets

- 2 tablespoons olive oil

- 1 lemon (sliced)

- 2 teaspoons dried thyme

- Salt and pepper to taste

Instructions:

1. Preheat the oven to 400°F (200°C).

2. Place cod fillets on a baking sheet.

3. Drizzle with olive oil, sprinkle with thyme, salt, and pepper.

4. Top each fillet with lemon slices.

5. Bake for about 15-20 minutes or until the fish is cooked through.

11.Lentil and Vegetable Curry

Ingredients:

- 1 cup dry lentils (rinsed)
- 1 can coconut milk
- 1 onion, chopped
- 2 carrots, diced
- 1 bell pepper, sliced
- 2 tablespoons curry powder
- 1 teaspoon turmeric
- 2 cloves garlic, minced
- Salt and pepper to taste

Instructions:

1. In a pot, combine lentils, coconut milk, onion, carrots, bell pepper, curry powder, turmeric, and garlic.

2. Bring to a simmer and cook until lentils are tender, about 25-30 minutes.

3. Season with salt and pepper to taste.

12.Egg and Vegetable Wrap

Ingredients:

- 4 whole-grain tortillas

- 4 eggs, beaten

- 1 cup mixed vegetables (spinach, tomatoes, mushrooms)

- 1/4 cup feta cheese, crumbled

- Salt and pepper to taste

Instructions:

1. In a skillet, scramble eggs until cooked through.

2. Add mixed vegetables and sauté until tender.

3. Warm tortillas and fill with the egg and vegetable mixture.

4. Sprinkle with feta cheese, season with salt and pepper.

13. Cucumber and Chickpea Salad

Ingredients:

- 2 cucumbers, diced

- 1 can chickpeas, drained and rinsed

- 1 cup cherry tomatoes, halved

- 1/4 cup red onion, finely chopped

- 2 tablespoons olive oil

- 1 tablespoon red wine vinegar

- Fresh mint leaves (optional)

- Salt and pepper to taste

Instructions:

1. In a large bowl, combine cucumbers, chickpeas, cherry tomatoes, and red onion.

2. In a small bowl, whisk together olive oil and red wine vinegar. Pour over the salad.

3. Toss gently to combine, add fresh mint leaves if desired.

4. Season with salt and pepper before serving.

14. Turkey and Vegetable Quinoa Bowl

Ingredients:

- 1 cup quinoa

- 1 lb ground turkey

- 1 zucchini, diced

- 1 bell pepper, chopped

- 1 cup broccoli florets

- 2 tablespoons soy sauce

- 1 tablespoon sesame oil

- 1 teaspoon ginger, grated

Instructions:

1. Cook quinoa according to package instructions.

2. In a skillet, cook ground turkey until browned. Add zucchini, bell pepper, and broccoli.

3. In a small bowl, mix soy sauce, sesame oil, and grated ginger. Pour over the turkey and vegetables.

4. Stir until well combined and serve over cooked quinoa.

15.Baked Apples with Cinnamon and Walnuts

Ingredients:

- 4 apples, cored and halved
- 1/4 cup chopped walnuts
- 2 tablespoons honey
- 1 teaspoon cinnamon

Instructions:

1. Preheat the oven to 375°F (190°C).
2. Place apple halves on a baking sheet.
3. In a bowl, mix chopped walnuts, honey, and cinnamon.
4. Spoon the mixture onto each apple half.
5. Bake for about 20-25 minutes or until apples are tender.

16.Salmon and Asparagus Foil Packets

Ingredients:

- 4 salmon fillets

- 1 bunch asparagus, trimmed

- 2 tablespoons olive oil

- 2 cloves garlic, minced

- 1 lemon, sliced

- Fresh dill for garnish

- Salt and pepper to taste

Instructions:

1. Preheat the oven to 400°F (200°C).

2. Place each salmon fillet on a piece of foil.

3. Arrange asparagus around each fillet, drizzle with olive oil, and sprinkle with minced garlic.

4. Season with salt and pepper, place lemon slices on top.

5. Seal the foil packets and bake for 15-20 minutes or until salmon is cooked through.

17.Cauliflower Rice Stir-Fry with Shrimp

Ingredients:

- 1 lb shrimp, peeled and deveined

- 1 head cauliflower, grated into rice-like texture

- 1 cup snap peas, trimmed

- 1 carrot, julienned

- 2 tablespoons low-sodium soy sauce

- 1 tablespoon sesame oil

- 1 teaspoon sriracha (optional)

- 2 green onions, chopped

Instructions:

1. In a wok or large skillet, stir-fry shrimp until pink and opaque. Set aside.

2. In the same pan, add cauliflower rice, snap peas, and carrot. Stir-fry until vegetables are tender.

3. Mix in cooked shrimp, soy sauce, sesame oil, and sriracha (if using).

4. Garnish with chopped green onions before serving.

18. Greek Yogurt Parfait with Berries and Almonds

Ingredients:

- 2 cups Greek yogurt

- 1 cup mixed berries (strawberries, blueberries, raspberries)

- 1/4 cup almonds, chopped

- 1 tablespoon honey

Instructions:

1. In a glass or bowl, layer Greek yogurt, mixed berries, and chopped almonds.

2. Drizzle honey over the top for sweetness.

3. Repeat the layers and finish with a sprinkle of almonds.

19.Chickpea and Vegetable Stir-Fry

Ingredients:

- 1 can chickpeas, drained and rinsed

- 2 cups broccoli florets

- 1 red bell pepper, sliced

- 1 cup snow peas, trimmed

- 2 tablespoons olive oil

- 2 tablespoons low-sodium soy sauce

- 1 tablespoon honey

- 1 teaspoon ginger, grated

Instructions:

1. In a wok or large skillet, sauté broccoli, bell pepper, and snow peas in olive oil until tender-crisp.

2. Add chickpeas to the vegetables and stir.

3. In a small bowl, mix soy sauce, honey, and grated ginger. Pour over the vegetables and chickpeas.

4. Stir until well coated and heated through.

20.Mango and Avocado Salsa with Grilled Chicken

Ingredients:

- 4 boneless, skinless chicken breasts

- 1 mango, diced

- 1 avocado, diced

- 1/4 cup red onion, finely chopped

- 1 jalapeño, minced (seeds removed for less heat)

- 1/4 cup cilantro, chopped

- Juice of 2 limes

- Salt and pepper to taste

Instructions:

1. Grill chicken breasts until fully cooked.

2. In a bowl, combine diced mango, avocado, red onion, jalapeño, cilantro, lime juice, salt, and pepper.

3. Serve grilled chicken topped with the mango and avocado salsa.

21. Baked Chicken and Vegetable Casserole

Ingredients:

- 4 boneless, skinless chicken thighs

- 1 cup cherry tomatoes, halved

- 1 zucchini, sliced

- 1 cup baby potatoes, halved

- 2 tablespoons olive oil

- 2 teaspoons Italian seasoning

- Salt and pepper to taste

Instructions:

1. Preheat the oven to 375°F (190°C).

2. Place chicken thighs in a baking dish.

3. Surround the chicken with cherry tomatoes, zucchini, and baby potatoes.

4. Drizzle with olive oil, sprinkle with Italian seasoning, salt, and pepper.

5. Bake for 30-35 minutes or until chicken is cooked through and vegetables are tender.

22.Caprese Salad with Balsamic Glaze

Ingredients:

- 2 cups cherry tomatoes, halved
- 1 cup fresh mozzarella, diced
- 1 bunch fresh basil leaves
- 2 tablespoons balsamic glaze
- Salt and pepper to taste

Instructions:

1. Arrange cherry tomatoes and mozzarella on a serving platter.
2. Tuck fresh basil leaves among the tomatoes and mozzarella.
3. Drizzle with balsamic glaze and season with salt and pepper.

23.Pumpkin and Lentil Soup

Ingredients:

- 1 cup dry red lentils (rinsed)

- 2 cups pumpkin, diced

- 1 onion, chopped

- 2 carrots, chopped

- 1 teaspoon cumin

- 1 teaspoon paprika

- 6 cups vegetable broth

- Salt and pepper to taste

Instructions:

1. In a pot, combine lentils, pumpkin, onion, carrots, cumin, paprika, and vegetable broth.

2. Bring to a boil, then reduce heat and simmer for 20-25 minutes or until lentils and vegetables are tender.

3. Season with salt and pepper to taste.

24.Sautéed Spinach with Garlic and Pine Nuts

Ingredients:

- 4 cups fresh spinach leaves

- 2 tablespoons olive oil

- 3 cloves garlic, minced

- 1/4 cup pine nuts

- Salt and pepper to taste

Instructions:

1. In a large skillet, heat olive oil over medium heat.

2. Add minced garlic and pine nuts, sauté until garlic is fragrant and pine nuts are golden.

3. Add fresh spinach and toss until wilted.

4. Season with salt and pepper before serving.

25.Sweet Potato and Black Bean Hash

Ingredients:

- 2 sweet potatoes, peeled and diced

- 1 can black beans, drained and rinsed

- 1 red bell pepper, diced

- 1 tablespoon olive oil

- 1 teaspoon cumin

- 1 teaspoon smoked paprika

- Salt and pepper to taste

Instructions:

1. In a skillet, heat olive oil over medium heat.

2. Add diced sweet potatoes, black beans, and red bell pepper.

3. Sprinkle with cumin, smoked paprika, salt, and pepper.

4. Sauté until sweet potatoes are tender and ingredients are well combined.

26.Turkey and Quinoa Stuffed Bell Peppers

Ingredients:

- 4 bell peppers, halved and seeds removed

- 1 lb ground turkey

- 1 cup cooked quinoa

- 1 cup black beans, drained and rinsed

- 1 cup corn kernels (fresh or frozen)

- 1 teaspoon cumin

- 1 teaspoon chili powder

- 1 cup tomato sauce

- Salt and pepper to taste

Instructions:

1. Preheat the oven to 375°F (190°C).

2. In a skillet, cook ground turkey until browned.

3. Mix in cooked quinoa, black beans, corn, cumin, chili powder, and half of the tomato sauce.

4. Fill each bell pepper half with the turkey and quinoa mixture.

5. Drizzle the remaining tomato sauce over the top.

6. Bake for 25-30 minutes or until peppers are tender.

27.Mushroom and Spinach Frittata

Ingredients:

- 8 eggs, beaten

- 1 cup mushrooms, sliced

- 2 cups fresh spinach leaves

- 1 onion, chopped

- 1/2 cup feta cheese, crumbled

- 2 tablespoons olive oil

- Salt and pepper to taste

Instructions:

1. Preheat the oven to 350°F (175°C).

2. In an oven-safe skillet, sauté mushrooms and onions in olive oil until softened.

3. Add fresh spinach and cook until wilted.

4. Pour beaten eggs over the vegetables, sprinkle with crumbled feta.

5. Cook on the stovetop for a few minutes, then transfer to the oven and bake until the eggs are set.

28.Roasted Brussels Sprouts with Cranberries and Pecans

Ingredients:

- 1 lb Brussels sprouts, trimmed and halved

- 1/2 cup dried cranberries

- 1/2 cup pecans, chopped

- 2 tablespoons olive oil

- 2 tablespoons balsamic vinegar

- Salt and pepper to taste

Instructions:

1. Preheat the oven to 400°F (200°C).

2. Toss Brussels sprouts, dried cranberries, and pecans with olive oil and balsamic vinegar.

3. Spread the mixture on a baking sheet.

4. Roast for 20-25 minutes or until Brussels sprouts are golden and caramelized.

29.Tuna and White Bean Salad

Ingredients:

- 2 cans tuna, drained

- 2 cans white beans, drained and rinsed

- 1 red onion, finely chopped

- 1 cucumber, diced

- 1/4 cup fresh parsley, chopped

- 2 tablespoons olive oil

- Juice of 1 lemon

- Salt and pepper to taste

Instructions:

1. In a large bowl, combine tuna, white beans, red onion, cucumber, and parsley.

2. Drizzle with olive oil and lemon juice.

3. Toss gently until well mixed.

4. Season with salt and pepper before serving.

30.Cinnamon-Baked Apples with Greek Yogurt

Ingredients:

- 4 apples, cored and sliced

- 1 tablespoon honey

- 1 teaspoon cinnamon

- 2 cups Greek yogurt

Instructions:

1. Preheat the oven to 375°F (190°C).

2. In a bowl, toss apple slices with honey and cinnamon.

3. Spread the apples on a baking sheet and bake for 15-20 minutes or until tender.

4. Serve the baked apples over Greek yogurt.

31.Lemon Garlic Shrimp with Zucchini Noodles

Ingredients:

- 1 lb shrimp, peeled and deveined

- 4 medium-sized zucchini, spiralized

- 2 tablespoons olive oil

- 3 cloves garlic, minced

- Juice of 2 lemons

- 1 teaspoon lemon zest

- Fresh parsley for garnish

- Salt and pepper to taste

Instructions:

1. In a skillet, heat olive oil over medium heat.

2. Add minced garlic and cook until fragrant.

3. Add shrimp to the skillet and cook until pink and opaque.

4. Toss in zucchini noodles, lemon juice, and lemon zest. Cook until the noodles are tender.

5. Season with salt and pepper, garnish with fresh parsley before serving.

32.Quinoa and Black Bean Stuffed Peppers

Ingredients:

- 4 bell peppers, halved and seeds removed

- 1 cup cooked quinoa

- 1 can black beans, drained and rinsed

- 1 cup corn kernels (fresh or frozen)

- 1 cup diced tomatoes

- 1 teaspoon cumin

- 1 teaspoon chili powder

- 1/2 cup shredded cheddar cheese

- Salt and pepper to taste

Instructions:

1. Preheat the oven to 375°F (190°C).

2. In a bowl, mix cooked quinoa, black beans, corn, diced tomatoes, cumin, and chili powder.

3. Fill each bell pepper half with the quinoa mixture.

4. Sprinkle shredded cheddar cheese on top.

5. Bake for 25-30 minutes or until peppers are tender and the cheese is melted.

33.Turmeric and Ginger Carrot Soup

Ingredients:

- 1 lb carrots, peeled and chopped
- 1 onion, chopped
- 2 tablespoons olive oil
- 1 teaspoon turmeric
- 1 teaspoon ginger, grated
- 4 cups vegetable broth
- Salt and pepper to taste
- Fresh cilantro for garnish

Instructions:

1. In a pot, sauté onions and carrots in olive oil until softened.
2. Add turmeric and ginger, stir to coat.
3. Pour in vegetable broth and bring to a simmer. Cook until carrots are tender.
4. Blend the soup until smooth.
5. Season with salt and pepper, garnish with fresh cilantro before serving.

34. Balsamic Glazed Chicken with Roasted Vegetables

Ingredients:

- 4 boneless, skinless chicken breasts

- 1 lb baby potatoes, halved

- 1 cup baby carrots

- 1 cup Brussels sprouts, trimmed and halved

- 3 tablespoons balsamic vinegar

- 2 tablespoons olive oil

- 1 tablespoon Dijon mustard

- Salt and pepper to taste

Instructions:

1. Preheat the oven to 400°F (200°C).

2. In a bowl, whisk together balsamic vinegar, olive oil, Dijon mustard, salt, and pepper.

3. Place chicken breasts and vegetables on a baking sheet.

4. Brush the balsamic mixture over the chicken and vegetables.

5. Roast for 25-30 minutes or until the chicken is cooked through and the vegetables are tender.

35.Mango Coconut Chia Pudding

Ingredients:

- 1/4 cup chia seeds

- 1 cup coconut milk

- 1 ripe mango, diced

- 1 tablespoon honey

- Shredded coconut for garnish

Instructions:

1. In a jar, mix chia seeds and coconut milk. Let it sit in the refrigerator for at least 2 hours or overnight.

2. Before serving, stir the chia pudding to ensure a smooth consistency.

3. Layer the chia pudding with diced mango.

4. Drizzle with honey and sprinkle shredded coconut on top.

36.Broccoli and Quinoa Casserole

Ingredients:

- 1 cup quinoa, cooked

- 2 cups broccoli florets

- 1 onion, finely chopped

- 1 cup shredded cheddar cheese

- 1 cup low-fat milk

- 2 tablespoons whole wheat flour

- 2 tablespoons olive oil

- Salt and pepper to taste

Instructions:

1. Preheat the oven to 375°F (190°C).

2. In a pan, sauté chopped onion and broccoli in olive oil until tender.

3. In a bowl, mix cooked quinoa, sautéed vegetables, and shredded cheddar cheese.

4. In a saucepan, whisk together milk and flour over medium heat until thickened.

5. Combine the quinoa mixture with the milk mixture and season with salt and pepper.

6. Transfer to a baking dish and bake for 25-30 minutes or until golden and bubbly.

37.Zesty Lemon Basil Chicken

Ingredients:

- 4 boneless, skinless chicken breasts

- Zest and juice of 2 lemons

- 1/4 cup fresh basil, chopped

- 2 tablespoons olive oil

- 2 cloves garlic, minced

- Salt and pepper to taste

Instructions:

1. Preheat the oven to 400°F (200°C).

2. In a bowl, mix lemon zest, lemon juice, chopped basil, minced garlic, olive oil, salt, and pepper.

3. Place chicken breasts in a baking dish and pour the lemon-basil mixture over them.

4. Bake for 25-30 minutes or until the chicken is cooked through.

38. Spaghetti Squash with Tomato and Basil Sauce

Ingredients:

- 1 spaghetti squash, halved and seeds removed

- 2 cups cherry tomatoes, halved

- 1/4 cup fresh basil, chopped

- 2 cloves garlic, minced

- 2 tablespoons olive oil

- Salt and pepper to taste

- Grated Parmesan cheese for topping

Instructions:

1. Preheat the oven to 375°F (190°C).

2. Place spaghetti squash halves, cut side down, on a baking sheet.

3. Bake for 30-40 minutes or until the squash is tender.

4. In a skillet, sauté cherry tomatoes, minced garlic, and chopped basil in olive oil until tomatoes are softened.

5. Use a fork to scrape the spaghetti squash into strands. Top with the tomato and basil sauce.

6. Season with salt and pepper, and sprinkle with grated Parmesan before serving.

39.Stuffed Portobello Mushrooms

Ingredients:

- 4 large Portobello mushrooms, stems removed

- 1 cup quinoa, cooked

- 1 cup spinach, chopped

- 1/2 cup feta cheese, crumbled

- 2 tablespoons balsamic glaze

- 2 tablespoons olive oil

- Salt and pepper to taste

Instructions:

1. Preheat the oven to 375°F (190°C).

2. Place Portobello mushrooms on a baking sheet.

3. In a bowl, mix cooked quinoa, chopped spinach, crumbled feta, and olive oil. Season with salt and pepper.

4. Stuff each mushroom with the quinoa mixture.

5. Bake for 20-25 minutes or until the mushrooms are tender.

6. Drizzle with balsamic glaze before serving.

40. Chilled Berry Soup

Ingredients:

- 2 cups mixed berries (strawberries, blueberries, raspberries)

- 1 cup plain yogurt

- 1/4 cup honey

- 1 tablespoon fresh mint, chopped

- 1/2 cup granola (optional)

Instructions:

1. In a blender, combine mixed berries, yogurt, honey, and mint. Blend until smooth.

2. Refrigerate the soup for at least 2 hours.

3. Serve chilled, garnished with additional berries and a sprinkle of granola if desired.

41.Baked Cod with Mediterranean Salsa

Ingredients:

- 4 cod fillets

- 1 cup cherry tomatoes, quartered

- 1/2 cup Kalamata olives, sliced

- 1/4 cup red onion, finely chopped

- 2 tablespoons fresh parsley, chopped

- 2 tablespoons olive oil

- 1 tablespoon balsamic vinegar

- Salt and pepper to taste

Instructions:

1. Preheat the oven to 400°F (200°C).

2. Place cod fillets on a baking sheet.

3. In a bowl, combine cherry tomatoes, olives, red onion, parsley, olive oil, and balsamic vinegar.

4. Spoon the Mediterranean salsa over the cod fillets.

5. Bake for 15-20 minutes or until the fish is cooked through.

42. Cauliflower and Broccoli Gratin

Ingredients:

- 1 head cauliflower, cut into florets

- 2 cups broccoli florets

- 1 cup shredded cheddar cheese

- 1/2 cup Parmesan cheese, grated

- 1 cup milk

- 2 tablespoons whole wheat flour

- 2 tablespoons butter

- 1 teaspoon Dijon mustard

- Salt and pepper to taste

Instructions:

1. Preheat the oven to 375°F (190°C).

2. Steam cauliflower and broccoli until just tender.

3. In a saucepan, melt butter over medium heat. Stir in flour and cook for 2 minutes.

4. Gradually whisk in milk until smooth and thickened.

5. Stir in Dijon mustard, shredded cheddar, and grated Parmesan until melted.

6. Combine the cheese sauce with steamed cauliflower and broccoli.

7. Transfer to a baking dish and bake for 20-25 minutes or until golden and bubbly.

43. Lemon Garlic Roasted Chicken Thighs

Ingredients:

- 4 chicken thighs, bone-in and skin-on

- Zest and juice of 1 lemon

- 3 cloves garlic, minced

- 2 tablespoons olive oil

- 1 teaspoon dried oregano

- 1 teaspoon paprika

- Salt and pepper to taste

Instructions:

1. Preheat the oven to 400°F (200°C).

2. In a bowl, mix lemon zest, lemon juice, minced garlic, olive oil, dried oregano, paprika, salt, and pepper.

3. Place chicken thighs on a baking sheet and brush with the lemon-garlic mixture.

4. Roast for 30-35 minutes or until the chicken is golden and cooked through.

44.Quinoa Salad with Roasted Vegetables

Ingredients:

- 1 cup quinoa, cooked

- 1 zucchini, diced

- 1 red bell pepper, diced

- 1 yellow bell pepper, diced

- 1 cup cherry tomatoes, halved

- 1/4 cup feta cheese, crumbled

- 2 tablespoons balsamic vinaigrette dressing

- Fresh basil for garnish

- Salt and pepper to taste

Instructions:

1. Preheat the oven to 400°F (200°C).

2. Toss diced zucchini, red bell pepper, and yellow bell pepper with olive oil, salt, and pepper.

3. Roast the vegetables for 20-25 minutes or until they are tender.

4. In a bowl, combine cooked quinoa, roasted vegetables, cherry tomatoes, and crumbled feta.

5. Drizzle with balsamic vinaigrette, toss gently, and garnish with fresh basil.

45.Minty Watermelon Salad

Ingredients:

- 4 cups watermelon, cubed

- 1 cucumber, sliced

- 1/4 cup fresh mint leaves, chopped

- 1/4 cup feta cheese, crumbled

- 2 tablespoons lime juice

- 1 tablespoon honey

- Salt to taste

Instructions:

1. In a large bowl, combine watermelon cubes, cucumber slices, and chopped mint.

2. In a small bowl, whisk together lime juice and honey.

3. Drizzle the dressing over the watermelon mixture and toss gently.

4. Sprinkle crumbled feta over the top and season with a pinch of salt.

46.Sesame Ginger Tofu Stir-Fry

Ingredients:

- 1 block extra-firm tofu, pressed and cubed

- 2 cups broccoli florets

- 1 red bell pepper, sliced

- 1 carrot, julienned

- 2 tablespoons sesame oil

- 3 tablespoons soy sauce

- 1 tablespoon rice vinegar

- 1 tablespoon fresh ginger, grated

- 1 tablespoon sesame seeds

- Green onions for garnish

- Brown rice for serving

Instructions:

1. In a wok or large skillet, heat sesame oil over medium-high heat.

2. Add cubed tofu and stir-fry until golden brown.

3. Add broccoli, red bell pepper, and julienned carrot. Cook until vegetables are tender-crisp.

4. In a small bowl, mix soy sauce, rice vinegar, and grated ginger. Pour over the tofu and vegetables.

5. Toss until everything is well coated. Sprinkle sesame seeds and garnish with chopped green onions.

6. Serve over cooked brown rice.

47.Mango and Avocado Quinoa Salad

Ingredients:

- 1 cup quinoa, cooked
- 1 mango, diced
- 1 avocado, diced
- 1/2 cup cherry tomatoes, halved
- 1/4 cup red onion, finely chopped
- 1/4 cup fresh cilantro, chopped
- Juice of 2 limes
- 2 tablespoons olive oil
- Salt and pepper to taste

Instructions:

1. In a large bowl, combine cooked quinoa, diced mango, diced avocado, cherry tomatoes, red onion, and cilantro.

2. In a small bowl, whisk together lime juice and olive oil. Pour over the salad.

3. Toss gently to combine. Season with salt and pepper to taste.

48.Honey Mustard Glazed Salmon

Ingredients:

- 4 salmon fillets

- 2 tablespoons Dijon mustard

- 2 tablespoons honey

- 1 tablespoon olive oil

- 1 teaspoon fresh dill, chopped

- Salt and pepper to taste

- Lemon wedges for serving

Instructions:

1. Preheat the oven to 400°F (200°C).

2. In a bowl, whisk together Dijon mustard, honey, olive oil, chopped dill, salt, and pepper.

3. Place salmon fillets on a baking sheet and brush with the honey mustard mixture.

4. Bake for 12-15 minutes or until the salmon is cooked through.

5. Serve with lemon wedges on the side.

49.Cabbage and Apple Slaw

Ingredients:

- 4 cups green cabbage, shredded

- 2 apples, julienned

- 1/2 cup Greek yogurt

- 2 tablespoons apple cider vinegar

- 1 tablespoon honey

- 1 teaspoon Dijon mustard

- Salt and pepper to taste

- Chopped walnuts for garnish

Instructions:

1. In a large bowl, combine shredded cabbage and julienned apples.

2. In a small bowl, whisk together Greek yogurt, apple cider vinegar, honey, Dijon mustard, salt, and pepper.

3. Pour the dressing over the cabbage and apples. Toss until well coated.

4. Garnish with chopped walnuts before serving.

50.Dark Chocolate and Berry Parfait

Ingredients:

- 2 cups Greek yogurt

- 1 cup mixed berries (strawberries, blueberries, raspberries)

- 1/4 cup dark chocolate chips

- 2 tablespoons honey

- Mint leaves for garnish

Instructions:

1. In a glass or bowl, layer Greek yogurt with mixed berries.

2. Sprinkle dark chocolate chips over each layer.

3. Drizzle honey on top for sweetness.

4. Repeat the layers and finish with a garnish of mint leaves.

51.Lemon Herb Quinoa with Roasted Vegetables

Ingredients:

- 1 cup quinoa, cooked

- 1 zucchini, sliced

- 1 yellow squash, sliced

- 1 red onion, thinly sliced

- 1 cup cherry tomatoes, halved

- 2 tablespoons olive oil

- Zest and juice of 1 lemon

- 2 tablespoons fresh herbs (such as parsley or basil), chopped

- Salt and pepper to taste

Instructions:

1. Preheat the oven to 400°F (200°C).

2. Toss zucchini, yellow squash, red onion, and cherry tomatoes with olive oil on a baking sheet.

3. Roast the vegetables for 20-25 minutes or until they are golden and tender.

4. In a large bowl, combine cooked quinoa, roasted vegetables, lemon zest, lemon juice, fresh herbs, salt, and pepper.

5. Mix well and serve as a flavorful and nutritious side dish.

52.Cilantro Lime Chicken Skewers

Ingredients:

- 1 lb chicken breast, cut into chunks

- Juice of 2 limes

- 1/4 cup fresh cilantro, chopped

- 2 tablespoons olive oil

- 1 teaspoon cumin

- 1 teaspoon paprika

- Salt and pepper to taste

- Wooden skewers, soaked in water

Instructions:

1. In a bowl, mix lime juice, chopped cilantro, olive oil, cumin, paprika, salt, and pepper to create the marinade.

2. Thread chicken chunks onto the soaked skewers.

3. Coat the chicken skewers with the marinade and let them marinate for at least 30 minutes.

4. Grill or broil the skewers for 8-10 minutes or until the chicken is cooked through.

5. Serve with additional lime wedges for squeezing over the top.

53.Roasted Garlic Mashed Cauliflower

Ingredients:

- 1 head cauliflower, cut into florets

- 2 cloves garlic, minced

- 2 tablespoons olive oil

- 1/4 cup Greek yogurt

- Salt and pepper to taste

- Chopped chives for garnish

Instructions:

1. Preheat the oven to 400°F (200°C).

2. Toss cauliflower florets and minced garlic with olive oil on a baking sheet.

3. Roast for 25-30 minutes or until the cauliflower is tender and golden.

4. Place the roasted cauliflower in a food processor. Add Greek yogurt, salt, and pepper.

5. Blend until smooth. Garnish with chopped chives before serving.

54. Black Bean and Corn Salsa

Ingredients:

- 1 can black beans, drained and rinsed

- 1 cup corn kernels (fresh or frozen)

- 1 red bell pepper, diced

- 1/4 cup red onion, finely chopped

- 1 jalapeño, minced (seeds removed for less heat)

- 2 tablespoons fresh cilantro, chopped

- Juice of 1 lime

- Salt and pepper to taste

Instructions:

1. In a bowl, combine black beans, corn, diced red bell pepper, red onion, minced jalapeño, and chopped cilantro.

2. Squeeze lime juice over the salsa and toss to combine.

3. Season with salt and pepper. Refrigerate for at least 30 minutes before serving.

4. Serve with whole-grain tortilla chips or as a topping for grilled chicken or fish.

55.Peach and Berry Smoothie Bowl

Ingredients:

- 1 cup frozen peaches

- 1/2 cup mixed berries (strawberries, blueberries, raspberries)

- 1/2 cup Greek yogurt

- 1/4 cup almond milk

- 1 tablespoon chia seeds

- Toppings: sliced almonds, shredded coconut, fresh berries

Instructions:

1. In a blender, blend frozen peaches, mixed berries, Greek yogurt, almond milk, and chia seeds until smooth.

2. Pour the smoothie into a bowl.

3. Top with sliced almonds, shredded coconut, and fresh berries.

4. Enjoy this refreshing and nutrient-packed smoothie bowl.

56.Salmon and Asparagus Foil Packets

Ingredients:

- 4 salmon fillets

- 1 bunch asparagus, trimmed

- 2 tablespoons olive oil

- 2 cloves garlic, minced

- Zest and juice of 1 lemon

- 1 teaspoon dill, chopped

- Salt and pepper to taste

Instructions:

1. Preheat the oven to 400°F (200°C).

2. Place each salmon fillet on a piece of aluminum foil.

3. Arrange asparagus around the salmon.

4. In a small bowl, mix olive oil, minced garlic, lemon zest, lemon juice, chopped dill, salt, and pepper.

5. Drizzle the mixture over the salmon and asparagus.

6. Seal the foil packets and bake for 15-20 minutes or until the salmon is cooked through.

57. Quinoa and Black Bean Stuffed Sweet Potatoes

Ingredients:

- 4 medium-sized sweet potatoes

- 1 cup quinoa, cooked

- 1 can black beans, drained and rinsed

- 1 cup corn kernels (fresh or frozen)

- 1 teaspoon cumin

- 1 teaspoon chili powder

- 1/2 cup salsa

- Fresh cilantro for garnish

Instructions:

1. Preheat the oven to 400°F (200°C).

2. Prick sweet potatoes with a fork and bake for 45-60 minutes or until tender.

3. In a bowl, mix cooked quinoa, black beans, corn, cumin, chili powder, and salsa.

4. Slice each sweet potato in half and fluff the insides with a fork.

5. Spoon the quinoa and black bean mixture over each sweet potato half.

6. Garnish with fresh cilantro before serving.

58.Greek Chicken Salad Wraps

Ingredients:

- 1 lb boneless, skinless chicken breasts, grilled and sliced

- 4 whole-grain wraps

- 1 cup cherry tomatoes, halved

- 1 cucumber, diced

- 1/2 cup Kalamata olives, sliced

- 1/2 cup feta cheese, crumbled

- Greek yogurt tzatziki sauce

- Fresh dill for garnish

Instructions:

1. In the center of each wrap, place sliced grilled chicken.

2. Add cherry tomatoes, diced cucumber, Kalamata olives, and crumbled feta.

3. Drizzle with Greek yogurt tzatziki sauce.

4. Sprinkle with fresh dill.

5. Wrap tightly and enjoy this flavorful Greek-inspired meal.

59.Cucumber Avocado Gazpacho

Ingredients:

- 2 cucumbers, peeled and chopped

- 2 ripe avocados, peeled and diced

- 1/2 cup fresh cilantro, chopped

- 1/4 cup red onion, finely chopped

- 2 cloves garlic, minced

- Juice of 2 limes

- 2 cups vegetable broth

- Salt and pepper to taste

- Greek yogurt for garnish (optional)

Instructions:

1. In a blender, combine chopped cucumbers, diced avocados, chopped cilantro, chopped red onion, minced garlic, lime juice, and vegetable broth.

2. Blend until smooth. Season with salt and pepper to taste.

3. Refrigerate for at least 2 hours before serving.

4. Garnish with a dollop of Greek yogurt if desired.

60.Almond Butter and Banana Overnight Oats

Ingredients:

- 1/2 cup rolled oats

- 1/2 cup almond milk

- 1 tablespoon almond butter

- 1 banana, sliced

- 1 tablespoon chia seeds

- 1 tablespoon honey

- Sliced almonds for topping

Instructions:

1. In a jar, combine rolled oats, almond milk, almond butter, banana slices, chia seeds, and honey.

2. Stir well, ensuring the oats are fully coated.

3. Refrigerate overnight.

4. Before serving, top with sliced almonds for a crunchy texture.

61. Turkey and Vegetable Stir-Fry

Ingredients:

- 1 lb ground turkey

- 2 cups broccoli florets

- 1 bell pepper, sliced

- 1 cup snap peas, trimmed

- 2 carrots, julienned

- 3 tablespoons low-sodium soy sauce

- 1 tablespoon hoisin sauce

- 1 tablespoon sesame oil

- 1 tablespoon ginger, minced

- 2 cloves garlic, minced

- Green onions for garnish

- Brown rice for serving

Instructions:

1. In a large skillet or wok, brown ground turkey over medium-high heat.

2. Add broccoli, bell pepper, snap peas, and carrots. Stir-fry until vegetables are tender-crisp.

3. In a small bowl, whisk together soy sauce, hoisin sauce, sesame oil, ginger, and garlic.

4. Pour the sauce over the turkey and vegetables. Stir until well coated and heated through.

5. Garnish with chopped green onions and serve over brown rice.

62.Caprese Salad with Grilled Chicken

Ingredients:

- 4 boneless, skinless chicken breasts, grilled

- 2 cups cherry tomatoes, halved

- 1 cup fresh mozzarella, diced

- 1/4 cup fresh basil, chopped

- 2 tablespoons balsamic glaze

- 2 tablespoons olive oil

- Salt and pepper to taste

Instructions:

1. Grill chicken breasts until fully cooked.

2. In a bowl, combine cherry tomatoes, fresh mozzarella, and chopped basil.

3. Slice grilled chicken and place it on top of the tomato and mozzarella mixture.

4. Drizzle with balsamic glaze and olive oil.

5. Season with salt and pepper to taste.

63.Miso-Glazed Eggplant with Quinoa

Ingredients:

- 2 large eggplants, sliced

- 1/4 cup white miso paste

- 2 tablespoons rice vinegar

- 1 tablespoon soy sauce

- 1 tablespoon sesame oil

- 1 tablespoon honey

- 1 cup quinoa, cooked

- Sesame seeds and sliced green onions for garnish

Instructions:

1. Preheat the oven to 400°F (200°C).

2. In a bowl, whisk together miso paste, rice vinegar, soy sauce, sesame oil, and honey.

3. Brush the eggplant slices with the miso mixture and place them on a baking sheet.

4. Roast for 20-25 minutes or until the eggplant is tender and caramelized.

5. Serve the miso-glazed eggplant over a bed of cooked quinoa.

6. Garnish with sesame seeds and sliced green onions.

64.Pesto Zoodles with Cherry Tomatoes

Ingredients:

- 4 medium zucchinis, spiralized into noodles

- 1 cup cherry tomatoes, halved

- 1/2 cup pesto sauce (store-bought or homemade)

- 1/4 cup pine nuts, toasted

- Grated Parmesan cheese for topping

Instructions:

1. In a large pan, sauté zucchini noodles over medium heat until just tender.

2. Add cherry tomatoes and cook for an additional 2-3 minutes.

3. Stir in pesto sauce and toss until the zoodles are well coated.

4. Toast pine nuts in a dry pan until golden.

5. Serve the pesto zoodles topped with toasted pine nuts and grated Parmesan.

65.Berry and Spinach Smoothie

Ingredients:

- 2 cups fresh spinach

- 1 cup mixed berries (strawberries, blueberries, raspberries)

- 1 banana

- 1/2 cup Greek yogurt

- 1 cup almond milk

- 1 tablespoon chia seeds

- Ice cubes (optional)

Instructions:

1. In a blender, combine fresh spinach, mixed berries, banana, Greek yogurt, almond milk, and chia seeds.

2. Blend until smooth.

3. Add ice cubes if desired and blend again until well combined.

4. Pour into a glass and enjoy this nutritious and refreshing smoothie.

66.Lentil and Vegetable Curry

Ingredients:

- 1 cup dried green lentils, rinsed and drained

- 1 onion, diced

- 2 carrots, diced

- 1 bell pepper, diced

- 1 zucchini, diced

- 3 cloves garlic, minced

- 1 can (14 oz) diced tomatoes

- 1 can (14 oz) coconut milk

- 2 tablespoons curry powder

- 1 teaspoon turmeric

- 1 teaspoon cumin

- Salt and pepper to taste

- Fresh cilantro for garnish

- Cooked brown rice for serving

Instructions:

1. In a large pot, sauté onion, carrots, bell pepper, and zucchini until softened.

2. Add minced garlic and cook for an additional minute.

3. Stir in curry powder, turmeric, and cumin, coating the vegetables.

4. Add lentils, diced tomatoes, and coconut milk. Season with salt and pepper.

5. Simmer for 25-30 minutes or until lentils are tender.

6. Serve over cooked brown rice, garnished with fresh cilantro.

67.Cauliflower and Chickpea Tacos

Ingredients:

- 1 head cauliflower, cut into florets

- 1 can (15 oz) chickpeas, drained and rinsed

- 2 tablespoons olive oil

- 1 teaspoon cumin

- 1 teaspoon smoked paprika

- 1/2 teaspoon chili powder

- 1/2 teaspoon garlic powder

- Corn tortillas

- Toppings: shredded lettuce, diced tomatoes, avocado slices, salsa

Instructions:

1. Preheat the oven to 400°F (200°C).

2. Toss cauliflower florets and chickpeas with olive oil, cumin, smoked paprika, chili powder, and garlic powder.

3. Spread the mixture on a baking sheet and roast for 25-30 minutes or until cauliflower is golden.

4. Warm corn tortillas and fill them with the roasted cauliflower and chickpea mixture.

5. Top with shredded lettuce, diced tomatoes, avocado slices, and salsa.

68.Mushroom and Spinach Quiche

Ingredients:

- 1 pie crust (store-bought or homemade)

- 1 cup mushrooms, sliced

- 2 cups fresh spinach

- 1 onion, diced

- 4 eggs

- 1 cup milk

- 1 cup shredded Gruyere or Swiss cheese

- Salt and pepper to taste

- Fresh thyme for garnish

Instructions:

1. Preheat the oven to 375°F (190°C).

2. In a skillet, sauté mushrooms, spinach, and onion until vegetables are softened.

3. In a bowl, whisk together eggs, milk, shredded cheese, salt, and pepper.

4. Place the pie crust in a pie dish. Spread the sautéed vegetables over the crust.

5. Pour the egg mixture over the vegetables.

6. Bake for 35-40 minutes or until the quiche is set and golden.

7. Garnish with fresh thyme before serving.

69.Sweet Potato and Black Bean Buddha Bowl

Ingredients:

- 2 medium sweet potatoes, cubed
- 1 can (15 oz) black beans, drained and rinsed
- 2 cups kale, chopped
- 1 avocado, sliced
- 1 cup cooked quinoa
- 2 tablespoons olive oil
- 1 teaspoon cumin
- 1 teaspoon paprika
- Salt and pepper to taste
- Tahini dressing for drizzling

Instructions:

1. Preheat the oven to 400°F (200°C).

2. Toss sweet potato cubes with olive oil, cumin, paprika, salt, and pepper.

3. Roast sweet potatoes for 25-30 minutes or until they are tender.

4. In a bowl, assemble the Buddha bowl with roasted sweet potatoes, black beans, kale, avocado slices, and cooked quinoa.

5. Drizzle with tahini dressing before serving.

70.Coconut Chia Seed Pudding with Mango

Ingredients:

- 1/4 cup chia seeds

- 1 cup coconut milk

- 1 tablespoon honey

- 1 teaspoon vanilla extract

- 1 ripe mango, diced

- Shredded coconut for topping

Instructions:

1. In a jar, mix chia seeds, coconut milk, honey, and vanilla extract. Refrigerate for at least 2 hours or overnight.

2. Before serving, stir the chia pudding to ensure a smooth consistency.

3. Layer the chia pudding with diced mango.

4. Sprinkle shredded coconut on top for added texture.

71.Spinach and Feta Stuffed Chicken Breast

Ingredients:

- 4 boneless, skinless chicken breasts

- 2 cups fresh spinach

- 1/2 cup feta cheese, crumbled

- 2 cloves garlic, minced

- 1 tablespoon olive oil

- 1 teaspoon dried oregano

- Salt and pepper to taste

- Lemon wedges for serving

Instructions:

1. Preheat the oven to 375°F (190°C).

2. In a skillet, sauté fresh spinach and minced garlic in olive oil until wilted.

3. Butterfly each chicken breast and stuff with sautéed spinach and crumbled feta.

4. Season the stuffed chicken breasts with dried oregano, salt, and pepper.

5. Place the stuffed chicken on a baking sheet and bake for 25-30 minutes or until the chicken is cooked through.

6. Serve with lemon wedges on the side.

72.Roasted Vegetable and Quinoa Stuffed Bell Peppers

Ingredients:

- 4 bell peppers, halved and seeds removed

- 1 cup quinoa, cooked

- 1 zucchini, diced

- 1 cup cherry tomatoes, halved

- 1/2 cup red onion, finely chopped

- 1 cup black beans, drained and rinsed

- 1 teaspoon cumin

- 1 teaspoon chili powder

- 1/2 cup shredded cheddar cheese

- Fresh cilantro for garnish

Instructions:

1. Preheat the oven to 375°F (190°C).

2. In a bowl, combine cooked quinoa, diced zucchini, halved cherry tomatoes, chopped red onion, black beans, cumin, and chili powder.

3. Stuff each bell pepper half with the quinoa mixture.

4. Top with shredded cheddar cheese.

5. Place stuffed peppers on a baking sheet and bake for 25-30 minutes or until the peppers are tender.

6. Garnish with fresh cilantro before serving.

73.Lemon Garlic Shrimp with Broccoli

Ingredients:

- 1 lb shrimp, peeled and deveined
- 2 cups broccoli florets
- 3 cloves garlic, minced
- Zest and juice of 1 lemon
- 2 tablespoons olive oil
- 1 teaspoon dried thyme
- Salt and pepper to taste
- Brown rice for serving

Instructions:

1. In a large skillet, heat olive oil over medium-high heat.

2. Add minced garlic and sauté until fragrant.

3. Add shrimp and cook until they turn pink.

4. Stir in broccoli florets, lemon zest, lemon juice, dried thyme, salt, and pepper.

5. Cook for an additional 5-7 minutes or until the broccoli is tender.

6. Serve the lemon garlic shrimp and broccoli over brown rice.

74.Avocado and Chickpea Salad

Ingredients:

- 2 cans (15 oz each) chickpeas, drained and rinsed

- 2 avocados, diced

- 1 cup cherry tomatoes, halved

- 1/4 cup red onion, finely chopped

- 1/4 cup fresh cilantro, chopped

- Juice of 2 limes

- 2 tablespoons olive oil

- Salt and pepper to taste

Instructions:

1. In a large bowl, combine chickpeas, diced avocados, halved cherry tomatoes, chopped red onion, and chopped cilantro.

2. In a small bowl, whisk together lime juice, olive oil, salt, and pepper.

3. Pour the dressing over the chickpea mixture and toss gently to combine.

4. Chill in the refrigerator for at least 30 minutes before serving.

75.Banana and Almond Butter Smoothie

Ingredients:

- 2 ripe bananas
- 2 tablespoons almond butter
- 1 cup Greek yogurt
- 1 cup almond milk
- 1 tablespoon honey
- Ice cubes (optional)

Instructions:

1. In a blender, combine ripe bananas, almond butter, Greek yogurt, almond milk, and honey.
2. Blend until smooth.
3. Add ice cubes if desired and blend again until well combined.
4. Pour into a glass and enjoy this creamy and satisfying smoothie.

76.Mediterranean Quinoa Salad

Ingredients:

- 1 cup quinoa, cooked
- 1 cucumber, diced
- 1 cup cherry tomatoes, halved
- 1/2 cup Kalamata olives, sliced
- 1/4 cup red onion, finely chopped
- 1/2 cup crumbled feta cheese
- 3 tablespoons olive oil
- 2 tablespoons balsamic vinegar
- 1 teaspoon dried oregano
- Salt and pepper to taste
- Fresh parsley for garnish

Instructions:

1. In a large bowl, combine cooked quinoa, diced cucumber, halved cherry tomatoes, sliced Kalamata olives, chopped red onion, and crumbled feta cheese.

2. In a small bowl, whisk together olive oil, balsamic vinegar, dried oregano, salt, and pepper.

3. Pour the dressing over the quinoa mixture and toss gently to coat.

4. Garnish with fresh parsley before serving.

77.Teriyaki Tofu Stir-Fry

Ingredients:

- 1 block extra-firm tofu, pressed and cubed
- 2 cups broccoli florets
- 1 bell pepper, sliced
- 1 carrot, julienned
- 1 cup snap peas, trimmed
- 3 tablespoons low-sodium teriyaki sauce
- 2 tablespoons soy sauce
- 1 tablespoon sesame oil
- 1 tablespoon rice vinegar
- 1 tablespoon sesame seeds
- Brown rice for serving

Instructions:

1. In a wok or large skillet, heat sesame oil over medium-high heat.

2. Add cubed tofu and stir-fry until golden brown.

3. Add broccoli, bell pepper, carrot, and snap peas. Cook until vegetables are tender-crisp.

4. In a small bowl, mix teriyaki sauce, soy sauce, rice vinegar, and sesame seeds.

5. Pour the sauce over the tofu and vegetables. Stir until well coated and heated through.

6. Serve over brown rice.

78. Cabbage and Apple Quinoa Salad

Ingredients:

- 2 cups red cabbage, shredded
- 1 apple, diced
- 1/2 cup walnuts, chopped
- 1/4 cup dried cranberries
- 1 cup quinoa, cooked
- 2 tablespoons apple cider vinegar
- 2 tablespoons olive oil
- 1 tablespoon Dijon mustard
- 1 tablespoon honey

- Salt and pepper to taste

Instructions:

1. In a large bowl, combine shredded red cabbage, diced apple, chopped walnuts, dried cranberries, and cooked quinoa.

2. In a small bowl, whisk together apple cider vinegar, olive oil, Dijon mustard, honey, salt, and pepper.

3. Pour the dressing over the salad and toss to combine.

4. Chill in the refrigerator for at least 30 minutes before serving.

79. Lemon Herb Baked Salmon

Ingredients:

- 4 salmon fillets
- Zest and juice of 1 lemon
- 2 tablespoons fresh parsley, chopped
- 1 tablespoon fresh dill, chopped
- 2 tablespoons olive oil
- 1 clove garlic, minced
- Salt and pepper to taste
- Lemon wedges for serving

Instructions:

1. Preheat the oven to 400°F (200°C).
2. In a small bowl, combine lemon zest, lemon juice, chopped parsley, chopped dill, olive oil, minced garlic, salt, and pepper.
3. Place salmon fillets on a baking sheet and brush with the lemon-herb mixture.
4. Bake for 12-15 minutes or until the salmon is cooked through.
5. Serve with lemon wedges on the side.

80.Green Smoothie Bowl

Ingredients:

- 2 cups spinach

- 1 frozen banana

- 1/2 avocado

- 1/2 cup pineapple chunks

- 1 cup coconut water

- Toppings: sliced kiwi, chia seeds, granola

Instructions:

1. In a blender, combine spinach, frozen banana, avocado, pineapple chunks, and coconut water.

2. Blend until smooth.

3. Pour the smoothie into a bowl and top with sliced kiwi, chia seeds, and granola.

4. Enjoy this vibrant and nutrient-packed green smoothie bowl.

Please note that the information provided here is for general knowledge and should not replace professional medical advice. If you have specific concerns or questions about Gallbladder Cancer, it's best to consult with a healthcare professional familiar with your medical history.

= THE END =

We appreciate you selecting this book! We hope your expectations were fulfilled or surpassed.

Please think about posting a review on social media if you liked our book. We value your opinion because it enables us to make improvements to our goods and services for future clients.

We want to thank you once more for your support and send our best to you.

www.ingramcontent.com/pod-product-compliance
Lightning Source LLC
Chambersburg PA
CBHW060949260726
48661CB00005B/1805